THE OUTCAST PHARMACIST

Desiring change in pharmacy education, professional standards, and bias in the healthcare industry

CONTENTS

This book is dedicated to the outcast pharmacist, those who want better for the profession of pharmacy, and pharmacists.

INTRODUCTION

Outcast*: a person or a group who has been rejected by society or a social group (Merriam-Webster).*

Those who work within the profession of pharmacy constantly pour out and give out knowledge, time, life, and wellbeing into others. Many pharmacists feel invisible until they are needed by society or other healthcare professionals. Now more than ever, we are seeing more burned out, stressed, and anxious pharmacists and realizing there are no advocacy groups that fight for their well-being.

As children, we never could say definitively what career path we saw ourselves working in, but we always enjoyed math, science, and helping others. Recognizing these strengths, our parents envisioned and had aspirations for us to become pharmacists. We didn't know the full scope of what pharmacy entailed, but we knew it did not involve having to deal with bodily fluids or having to touch patients. In addition, we always heard that this profession would allow individuals to become doctors within their early twenties and earn a six-figure income. So, when people asked what we wanted to go to college for, pharmacy became an automatic response.

Halfway through pharmacy school, we felt like we made a mistake and did not have anyone we could speak with about it. We felt as if we were placed in a box and filled with a hunger of wanting more for the profession. Our interest grew in wanting to learn more about the behind-the-scenes decisions, processes, systems, and policies that determined how the profession of pharmacy functions. The courses that interested us the most were some of the least emphasized in pharmacy education: management and leadership, public health, and pharmacoeconomics. In practice, we found that these subjects influence professional outcomes either in an effective or ineffective manner.

Furthermore, as we were going through our pharmacy program, we kept being told by professors and preceptors (those that provide hands-on training within diverse fields of pharmacy required for graduation) that clinical pharmacy is the future of the profession. They advised that not to be a part of this movement would deem us unsuccessful or unattractive to employers. We quickly learned that to be exclusively clinical meant that we likely would still end up in a narrow path of work. A position as the pharmacy director of a clinic or hospital would be the ceiling of professional success.

By grace, we are practicing pharmacy as a short-termed career. However, we are grateful for the trials we have experienced, because they further refined us as people and as professionals. Undoubtedly, our verbal and written communication, interpersonal skills, cultural responsiveness, and adversity navigation are now sharper than they would have been if not for our careers in pharmacy.

Therefore, we want to clarify the intentions and goals we have set for this book. We will share the day-in the-life experiences of some pharmacists as related to current issues in the industry. We will inform those inside and outside the healthcare field about what pharmacy is. We will recount some of the important experiences we have had and stories we have heard from other pharmacists. Lastly, we will illuminate the spirit of resentment that has entered into the field of pharmacy. This resentment has kept many pharmacists and aspiring pharmacists in mental, physical, or financial bondage.

The profession is plummeting right now. It will be a *breaking* point or *breakthrough* point, depending on how all stakeholders take action. Based on our knowledge and experiences, we are hopeful for the latter. Still, a breakthrough only happens when we acknowledge what is breaking down. The most active advocacy groups are fighting to expand the role of pharmacists, but there is not a clear focus on workload issues, especially within the community, retail, and production/packaging settings.

It is our hope that this book will enlighten those who are not knowledgeable of the specialized healthcare profession of pharmacy. We hope to shed light on common challenges pharmacists may face and to discuss the silent pain that many pharmacists often suppress to maintain their livelihood. The spirit of resentment that we mentioned can be resolved, but only after we unearth and resolve the problems that birthed it. We hope that this book is a first step toward something all pharmacists value: healing.

CHAPTER 1:
WHAT IS A PHARMACIST?

Pharmacist: someone who is a healthcare professional licensed to engage in pharmacy, with duties including dispensing prescription drugs, monitoring drug interactions, administering vaccines, and counseling patients regarding the effects and proper usage of drugs and dietary supplements (Merriam-Webster).

Our main objective here is to establish an understanding of the basic tenets of pharmacy. We will explore where some pharmacists work within the profession and what some pharmacists' duties and tasks are. Lastly, we will recognize a few key skills and qualities of pharmacists that are transferrable for employment within other fields such as education, communications, administration, business, marketing, finance, and risk management roles.

So many are underinformed about what pharmacy is, what a pharmacist actually does, the skill sets of a pharmacist, and all of the places where a pharmacist can work. Some people have no idea that pharmacists are doctors. Everyone who has obtained a doctor of pharmacy degree, also known as a PharmD, is a doctor. A PharmD is not akin to a PhD, despite that being a popular belief. A PhD is a doctor of philosophy, and it can be obtained within various disciplines such as music, education, public health, business, art, criminology, social work, toxicology, and more.

Pharmacists utilize so many strengths and disseminate knowledge, which can be classified as soft skills and interpersonal skills. These encompass being great problem-solvers, analytical and critical thinkers, multi-taskers, and listeners. Pharmacists also must be very detail-oriented, be able to educate or provide complex information to others, and be excellent with numbers and calculations.

These are just a few of the required skills, but the point we want to make is that pharmacists are excellent at doing things many may have never thought of due to a lack of knowledge of the profession. A pharmacist is also the most visible healthcare professional in the eye of the public due to the community or retail settings. Community or retail pharmacists are most visible due to their accessibility and no need to make or schedule an appointment time to receive a free consultation during the midst of their workflow.

A pharmacist can work in various settings, but the most common places that the general public is aware of are the community or chain retail and hospital settings. The other settings are hidden jewels, depending on whom you ask. Below is a list of the various professional settings for pharmacists provided by the American Pharmacists Association (APhA):
1. Academia: Clinical Practice
2. Academia: Economic, Social, and Administrative Sciences (ESAS)
3. Academia: Pharmaceutical Sciences
4. Ambulatory Care
5. Association Management

6. Chain Community Pharmacy: Management
7. Clinical Specialists
8. Community Health Center (CHC)
9. Compounding Pharmacy
10. Contract Research Organization
11. Corporate Management
12. Government/Federal Pharmacy
13. Home Health Care
14. Health System Pharmacy: Inpatient
15. Health System Pharmacy: Outpatient
16. Independent Community Pharmacy
17. Long Term Care
18. Mail Service
19. Managed Care
20. Medical Communications/Drug Information
21. Nuclear Pharmacy
22. Office-based Medication Management
23. Pharmaceutical Industry: Medical Liaison
24. Pharmaceutical Industry: Research and Development (R&D)
25. Pharmaceutical Industry Sales and Marketing
26. Pharmacy Benefit Management (PBM)
27. Pharmacy Law/Regulatory Affairs/Public Policy
28. Specialty Pharmacy

To further understand a pharmacist's role within these settings, please conduct further research through the American Pharmacist Association (APhA) website or other industry-recognized sources.

We want to pause here to recognize pharmacy technicians. Despite often being overlooked, pharmacy technicians are valuable assets to the profession. They are dynamic in regards to the operations of a pharmacy working efficiently and effectively. Many pharmacists previously worked as pharmacy technicians and, therefore, they understand the profession from various workflow perspectives. Amazing "pharm techs" have assisted us numerous times in numerous ways that we will appreciate forever. Bear them in mind as we continue defining the roles and experiences of pharmacists.

Even though the accessibility is there for consultations in the retail and community settings, they are predominantly brief due to production work that must be completed for the attaining of time and volume metrics. For those who do not know, production work within a pharmacy takes place when a prescription is received in a pharmacy electronically (e-script), via telephonically (written), or as a paper prescription. These versions of the prescription must first be typed. Typing must take place in the correct patient's profile. A patient's prescription insurance has to be located or identified next for accurate pricing, or there may be a coupon or patient assistance discount that has to be identified. Lastly, the prescription must be billed to the correct doctor or provider.

The next process after the typed prescription has been processed for pricing is for it to be verified for validity and correctness. This is when the pharmacy can create and print a label for the vial, box, stock bottle, or other container. The prescription is then filled or packaged with the correct medication according to the specified quantity, strength, day supply, and dosage form. It is then reviewed in a final check for completion within an allotted time frame. The process is pretty comparable to that of a fast-food restaurant.

Some pharmacists review anywhere from fifty to thousands of prescriptions per day. All pharmacists have to meet what is called a verified-by promise time, filled-by promise time, or a similarly titled metric. These metrics do not take into account understaffed facilities, patient phone calls, doctor's office phone calls, insurance hiccups, foot traffic, patients that may come in for a vaccination(s), consultations, refills, prescription transfers, or those who bring in a paper prescription(s). The topic of pharmacists' additional tasks will be discussed further in Chapter 3.

One of the most common recommendations pharmacists use to reduce the likelihood of medication errors and harm is to review the "five rights." Medication errors and risks are prevented much more often when the five rights are completed. The five rights are as follows:

1. the right patient
2. the right drug
3. the right dose
4. the right route
5. the right time

The tradition of filling prescriptions within an allotted time frame is quite horrifying when all factors are considered. Medications have the potential to cause harm, and in some cases, death. Timing when a prescription should be filled and verified invites errors to occur that can be life-threatening to a consumer. Potential errors also can be life-altering to anyone involved within the prescription process, because they may lose their pharmacist license, job, career prospects, or freedom.

CHAPTER 2:
HOW DOES ONE BECOME A
PHARMACIST?

We established in Chapter 1 that a pharmacist is a doctor. Now, let's delve into the rigorous educational training and internship hours required of them. One becomes a pharmacist by completing, on average, six to eight years of schooling. Students who enter college with the intention of becoming a pharmacist undergo two years or longer of prerequisites without attaining a bachelor's degree, then they apply to a three-year or four-year pharmacy program. The second most common approach is to graduate with a bachelor's degree or a bachelor's and a master's degree before applying to a three-year or four-year pharmacy program.

Along with what may become a maximum of ten years in school, there are entry exams, internships, comprehensive exams, and licensure exams to consider. Some pharmacy schools require their applicants to take a pre-entry exam called the PCAT. Its status is comparable to other rigorous entry exams, such as the MCAT exam for medical school or the LSAT for law school. For programs that do not require their applicants to take the PCAT, they often require their students to take and pass their school's comprehensive exit exam in order to graduate.

As a pharmacy intern in a traditional four-year program, candidates are referred to as **P1** - 1st year pharmacy student, **P2** - 2nd year pharmacy student, **P3** - 3rd year pharmacy student, or **P4** - 4th year pharmacy student. During the P1 through P3 years, students are required to obtain exposure to the retail/community and hospital pharmacy settings. This stage is called Introductory Pharmacy Practice Experience (IPPE). Typically, only one month of hands-on training is required with supervision from a pharmacist.

Within pharmacy schools in the state of Florida, a pharmacy student-candidate becomes a "pharmacy intern" during their P1 through P4 years. The state defines a pharmacy intern as a person who is currently registered in and attending a duly accredited college or school of pharmacy, or a graduate of such a school or college of pharmacy, and who is duly and properly registered with the department of health as provided for under its rules.

During this phase, pharmacy interns realize that sacrifices must be made. Time spent with loved ones may be limited, vacations may have to be planned far in advance, and extracurricular activities may be paused or adjusted because of the amount of studying required. Even some friendships or relationships are ended due to the lack of understanding for the need to prioritize studying.

P1 through P3 years mostly consist of didactic work or lecturing and studying. Unfortunately, during these years, pharmacy students do not know or learn much about the actual practice of pharmacy, unless they sought after and received a pharmacy intern position or an employment opportunity on their own. These roles are often difficult to obtain, the hours for work are minimal, and opportunities are limited to a few areas within the profession.

During the P4 year, pharmacy students must complete what is called pharmacy rotations or their Advanced Pharmacy Practice Experience (APPE). This timeframe is allotted to expose students to various pharmacy settings. In our experience, we had no say in which opportunities we would have liked to experience. However, we both had the opportunity of a rotational experience within the U.S. Food and Drug Administration (FDA) due to a selection process. We gained valuable knowledge of policies that regulated drug marketing, development, processes, and systems.

During rotations, we and many others experienced preceptors that spoke in a condescending manner and consistently interrogated us as to what our goals were post-graduation. Most of them assumed what we liked and disliked instead of teaching us their role and giving guidance on what is to be expected as a registered pharmacist. Most preceptors we encountered enjoyed the power trip or authoritative aspect of their role, but they did not understand the importance of teaching and instilling knowledge.

Some ways to address this problem is to have an unbiased advocate involved in the experience that ensures the well-being of pharmacy students within each pharmacy school's program. Students should be able to speak up about their concerns. Yet, we have witnessed students being put to shame, harassed, or threatened with delayed graduation simply for using their voices.

The need for unbiased advocates is abundantly clear in cases when the same complaint has been made several times. Every such concern should be documented and addressed. Unfortunately, many preceptors are often not equipped with effective teaching skills or coaching strategies. Most P4 students just want to do their work, learn, and go home to study for their licensure exams, but an ineffective preceptor will inhibit these students' success. Currently, the preceptor-intern relationship remains largely unsupervised and unchecked.

After a pharmacy student/pharmacy intern has completed all of their rotations and has passed other requirements set forth by their program, they become pharmacy graduates (also called "pharmacy graduate interns"). In order to become a licensed pharmacist or registered pharmacist (RPh), there are requirements that pharmacy graduates must meet. First, they must apply and pay a fee to register as a healthcare professional with their state's department of health. They must register with the National Association of Boards of Pharmacy (NABP), pay all board exam fees, and pass all board exams within an allotted number of attempts in a specified timeframe.

On average, pharmacy graduates take two or three exams, depending on the laws of the state in which they will practice. The two main exams pharmacy graduates take are the North American Pharmacist Licensure Examination (NAPLEX) and the Multistate Pharmacy Jurisprudence Examination (MPJE). Once these particular exams are completed, there are many others that pharmacists can take to further specialize within a particular disease state(s) or area of pharmacy practice.

As previously stated, receiving a license and employment as a registered pharmacist is contingent upon passing the required exams. The NAPLEX is a 6-hour exam and 200 questions are used to calculate exam results. The MPJE is a 2.5-hour exam and 100 questions are used to calculate exam results. Both exams are computerized and facilitated by a proctor. Graduates must spend a significant amount of time finding a location, date, and time to take these exams. Due to limited availability, some graduates schedule their exams in distant cities or states. With these factors in mind, we advise graduates to register several weeks in advance of their ideal testing time.

A pharmacist can be licensed to practice in as many states as they would like, but they must pay fees, pass all required exams, meet certain qualifications, and complete continuing education courses also known as CEs. Keeping one's license valid in multiple states can be tedious. Some states require that certain CE topics are reviewed for each licensure renewal period. For example, the state of Florida requires that pharmacists take two hours of "medication errors" courses and two hours of "controlled substances" courses every biennial period.

Every pharmacist's license must be renewed biennially. Some pharmacists have to pay to take their continuing education courses and some pharmacists' employers pay for their CE courses. Nevertheless, during every renewal period, a pharmacist has to pay a fee in order to have their license up-to-date, which allows them to continue in their respective pharmacy practice.

CHAPTER 3:
THE SILENT PAIN

Knowing the primary functions and credentials of a pharmacists are important precursors to understanding the current sentiments of pharmacists. We will now discuss what many pharmacists have felt, are currently feeling, and will continue to experience if the profession does not advance in its ways to advocate for pharmacists' well-being. Again, not all pharmacists agree with or experience the social-emotional concerns we will share. We are speaking for those who do. We refer to their collective truths as *the silent pain*.

The silent pain is experienced as long-suffering. Many do not understand why pharmacists bear this pain because they only know about the stereotypical financial gain of the professional. Most outsiders do not know the physical and psychological trauma pharmacists experience. Moreover, it is understandably difficult for those who academically, morally, or financially supported an individual's journey to becoming a pharmacist to witness such a drastic shift.

Therefore, pharmacists' desires to quit or to move on to a totally different sector can birth a variety of fears. There is the fear of identifying and pursuing a new career. There is the fear that their new profession will not offer the financial support that their family needs. There is the fear that family and friends will make them feel as if they are a quitter or that they do not know what they want to do in life. We certainly have been there. Even when a pharmacist wants a way out, they may not know there is one. They may lack the education or support needed to make the transition. So, they continue to suffer silently.

This silent pain causes burnout, distress, and exhaustion, resulting in a lack of passion for the work they do. It often appears or manifests as depression, frustration, aggravation, withdrawal, and emotional numbness. Pharmacists in silent pain carry the burden of not speaking their untold truth, and it is a heavy one to bear. The silent pain mirrors employee burnout in other sectors, and, within healthcare, it should be of ultimate national concern. Patients' lives are in the hands of overworked healthcare professionals. We are thankful for the trust placed in us and our colleagues in white coats, but we are not machines. We are humans being forced to adhere to superhuman standards.

Job burnout or occupational burnout: a type of work-related stress, a state of physical, mental, or emotional exhaustion that also involves a sense of reduced accomplishment and loss of personal identity. Accompanied by a lack of motivation, frustration, a slip in job performance, not taking full care of oneself (Merriam-Webster).

Emotionally exhausted: emotionally worn-out and drained as a result of accumulated stress from one's work life or a combination of both (Merriam-Webster).

Alert fatigue or alarm fatigue: occurs when one is exposed to a large number or frequently being alarmed/notified by alerts. Over time one can become desensitized to such alerts/alarms and miss important suggestions resulting in unwanted results and effects (Merriam-Webster).

Overworked: *having to work beyond their capacity or strength, possibility to cause physical and/or mental distress in the process (Merriam-Webster). Leaves room for error.*

Distress: *pain or suffering affecting the body, a bodily part, or the mind, a painful situation (Merriam-Webster).*

Understaffed: *having few staff members to operate effectively, safely, and efficiently (Merriam-Webster).*

Regret: *an emotion of feeling sad, repentant, or disappointed over something that has happened or from a loss or missed opportunity (Merriam-Webster).*

Eating disorders (gluttony): *excessive eating or a (**loss of appetite**): not eating or drinking water to stay well-nourished (Merriam-Webster). Many metabolic disorders have occurred in the lives of pharmacists unconsciously.*

Physical, physiological, and psychological distress: *development of health conditions due to dehydration, poor appetite/nutritional intake resulting in depression, obesity, high blood pressure, knee/leg/back and pain (musculoskeletal pain/disorders), carpal tunnel, blood clotting, and many others (Merriam-Webster).*

As floater pharmacists, the commute can be brutal or enjoyable. One's feelings about the commute greatly depends on the distance one is required to travel for work and the hours needed to labor for that day. Speaking from our own experiences as floater pharmacists within the retail/community settings, schedules may be inconsistent and required travel may be up to 50 to 100 miles in one direction for either a 12-hour, 8-hour, or 6-hour shift. This typically is not mentioned in pharmacy school. Floater pharmacists also have to adjust to each pharmacy location's environment, coming in with the objective to keep the pharmacy in order while filling in for the day.

Every pharmacy flows differently, and the technicians who are assigned to a pharmacy vary greatly as well. We have experienced technicians who complicate floater pharmacists' jobs with inefficiency or unprofessionalism. We have also worked with technicians who seamlessly collaborate with floaters just as if their pharmacy manager or staff pharmacist were there. As we mentioned in Chapter 1, pharmacy technicians are essential to the operation of a pharmacy, so their conduct holds a significant impact.

The variations floater pharmacists experience can be frustrating, especially when others with longevity in their roles or positions are resistant to change. When people do not want to adjust and are stuck in their ways, there is room for error. Further, schedulers may just place floater pharmacists into a spot so a body can be present, but they may not take into consideration important factors. The environment, consistency, and volume are critical to a pharmacist's ability to work smoothly and effectively.

Many within the general public do not know that lunch breaks for pharmacists are not mandatory. Some states or counties have mandated a 30-minute break for pharmacists, but they cannot leave the premises, because that deems the pharmacy closed by law. Some organizations or companies have not addressed this because pharmacists are often classified as salaried employees. As such, taking a lunch break or not is at the discretion of the pharmacist, which is a lose-lose scenario. If pharmacists decide to use the restroom, take a 15-minute break, or even a brief pause, they cannot meet their required metrics. While the policy fight for a mandatory work-free lunch break is gaining some prevalence, raising public awareness will increase the likelihood of change.

Every second, every minute, and every hour is critical to one who is a retail/community pharmacist. Current standards are prioritizing metrics over patients. A tired or distressed employee makes an incompetent healthcare professional. Many that determine and uphold pharmacy metric requirements are not practicing pharmacists. Some are ex-pharmacists in leadership roles that do not advocate for those they left behind. The understaffing and unrealistic demands required of a pharmacist within their workday takes life away from a caring and empathetic practitioner.

Being underappreciated for what we commit to is another source of silent pain. We have witnessed many pharmacists take on more than others just to keep the operations of a pharmacy afloat. Some give up time with family and loved ones because of the fear of losing their job. It is especially painful to recall the injustices leveraged against women in the field. One of our colleagues was told that she must figure out a plan to keep the pharmacy she manages running efficiently and thriving while she was out for maternity leave.

Furthermore, the addiction, dependency, and diversion of many dispensed prescriptions receives a forced blind eye and burdens many pharmacists. As pharmacists, many know that they are unwilfully aiding those with drug addiction, dependency, and abuse disorders. This frustration goes unnoticed because, at the end of the day, the prescriptions have to be filled. The current structure revolves around making profit, even if those profits are made on the backs of vulnerable addicts.

This chapter is not intended to discourage those who aspire to work in this field, but to share unfiltered experiences that indicate what can take place if reform is not implemented. Such information was not given to us in an academic setting. We had to acquire it through our years of didactic training and career experiences. Aspiring pharmacists deserve to know the wide range of circumstances and requirements they will encounter as professionals, which is one of our major motivations here.

Many pharmacists enjoy their roles and impact on society as frontline healthcare professionals. Speaking about the silent pain of our suffering colleagues is not an affront to our satisfied colleagues. It is the very opposite. The reforms we are calling for support the well-being and professionalism of all pharmacists, regardless of their current sentiments. Our advocacy is about pharmacists being able to meet their basic human needs at work and patients being able to trust that their lives are in the best hands.

One of the most critical layers to pharmacists' silent pain stems from financial bondage. The student loan debt of the average pharmacist is astronomical. Juxtaposing student loan debt with a pharmacist's salary, many pharmacists decide not to leave the profession. After attaining or accumulating a certain amount financially, or earning a salary that is uncommon in other fields, taking a pay cut for the sake of peace is still too life-altering for some to risk. So, some pharmacists encourage pharmacy students and peers to take into consideration and to thoroughly spend time thinking about why they would want to pursue pharmacy as their career field.

Lastly, the general public is not aware of how often a pharmacist has to work in a pharmacy alone. When a pharmacy technician is out for a lunch break, a pharmacy technician calls out, or the last 1-3 hours before closing, pharmacists often work solo. Companies often attribute this to slow workflow or to lacking the budget to pay a technician, totally disregarding the fact that it is unsafe for one person (the pharmacist) to be working a drive-thru window, registers, phones, and walk-ins simultaneously.

Safety measures or policies should be set in place to support employees when working alone. Providing pharmacists with breaks and safety measures is a simple and doable ask. Our proposal is that two employees always close a pharmacy together. Further, employees having the same break times would help to prevent errors and unsafe situations. In addition to the everyday obnoxious patient, we have experienced or witnessed death threats, threatening notes left on cars, robberies, and murders.

CHAPTER 4:
SOME WANT OUT

Working as a pharmacist is not for the weak, but for the indestructible. In the field of pharmacy, harassment and condescension are widely experienced. Many times, pharmacists endure physical hostility and abrasive comments from patients, caregivers, co-workers, managers, directors, and other healthcare professionals. It occurs for a number of reasons, but we hope that through this book and other awareness efforts that individuals will be more graceful and understanding.

We have experienced or witnessed remarks such as, "How do you not know this?" or "Sure, just do it however you want, you are a pharmacist." Many pharmacists and other professionals that have been practicing for years often forget that they were once a new hire and did not know all of the things they know now at the beginning of their careers. Some do not even consider that the pharmacist they are mistreating may be a floater pharmacist that is unfamiliar with the operation of that particular setting.

It is sad when we hear patients state that they do not know what medications they are taking and why they are taking them. Patients often think that pharmacists know exactly why they are taking a particular medication, but we can know only a possibility as to why they are taking it. This lack of information is due to several factors, including limited access and interoperability of health information technology systems. Unless a community pharmacy or ambulatory care pharmacy has been given access to look at a patient's chart or electronic medical record (EMR), the information is inaccessible to pharmacists.

Further, within a retail or community pharmacy setting, redundant and repetitive tasks are done every day. Some pharmacists who stay for many years do so partly because of this consistency. On the other hand, those who desire to expand their experiences in the administrative, educational, financial, and technological aspects of healthcare become exhausted, disinterested, unsatisfied, bored, and unfulfilled.

These outcast pharmacists, which we are, often become invisible healthcare professionals--only needed when a medication is involved or when a free consultation is requested. As of the COVID-19 pandemic and vaccine rollout, we are appreciated occasionally, if we are not mistaken to be a nurse or medical doctor. We certainly respect and value all of our healthcare colleagues, and we wish the same level of regard for pharmacists.

What exactly do we mean by *some want out*? We know others like us who want out of this traditional box that pharmacists are placed in by society and the healthcare industry. Some want to be completely out of the field of pharmacy, some want out of the traditional way things are done, and others just want out from their current role or employer. These reasons may be seen as either negative or positive among seasoned pharmacists, depending on whom you ask.

People may wonder why someone would give up a career that pays, on average, $50+ an hour. However, most recent graduates or newly hired pharmacists no longer get paid the stereotypical six-figure salary. This is due to budget cuts that result in reduced hours (32 hours or less per week) and reduced pay. When we review pharmacists' historical salaries and bonuses, their employers are now saving millions of dollars in labor costs. This does not account for potential budget redistributions that safeguard companies or organizations from legal conflicts, disputes, and insurance claims.

Cutting eight pharmacists that earn $125,000 annually saves a company or an organization $1,000,000.
If we apply this calculation to every county, city, and state making these budgets cuts, it is easy to discover a major cause of job shortages for pharmacists despite a presumably oversaturated market. This debunks the popular "six years six figures" concept that historically recruited aspiring pharmacists.

A common belief within the profession is that the market is saturated and it is difficult to find employment that is truly fulfilling. Many pharmacists take a job due to overwhelming student loan debt, the need to support a family, and simply for sustaining a living. These factors discourage thousands of pharmacists from pursuing other careers or entrepreneurship.

The degree of a pharmacist (PharmD) is not recognized within other industries or even seen as versatile within healthcare as in the case of, for example, a nursing degree (RN, ARNP, etc.). We believe that pharmacists would be excellent at enhancing continuous quality improvement measures, reviewing data to improve economic growth and development, and within administrative roles to help healthcare systems and processes become more efficient (this will be addressed in Chapter 5).

Some pharmacists go back to school for master's degrees in hopes of entering the business (pharmaceutical industry or managed care) and technological aspects of pharmacy and healthcare. Others pursue careers in academia. Some return to school and become a two-time doctor (mind blowing, right?). We know and have seen pharmacists become lawyers (Juris Doctorate/JD), medical doctors (MD), dentists (DMD/DDS), or experts within another discipline (Doctor of Philosophy/PhD).

We know that many pharmacists decide to take these avenues out in order to enhance healthcare overall and to pursue a better quality of life for themselves. After witnessing so many harrowing circumstances firsthand, many pharmacists ultimately seek to prevent patients from having to receive a prescribed medication for a preventable disease (i.e., diabetes, high blood pressure, high cholesterol, etc.). Trending toward prevention can be summarized as improved or optimal health outcomes.

Improving health outcomes also leads to a correlation in improved quality of life. Drugs do not cure, but they may treat, maintain, or sustain. As pharmacist, we know that drugs treat symptoms and aid in regulating the body into homeostasis. We are not against the use of prescription drugs, but preventable inflammatory diseases and chronic disease states (diabetes, hypertension, and high cholesterol) are often due to one's social determinants of health. The same is true of some mental illnesses. Some of these determinants are entirely preventable.

We believe that if equitable policies and programs were put in place, premature and preventable deaths would decrease. There would be an improved quality of life, and a decrease in the overall U.S. healthcare expenditure. Pharmacists can lead the way to this new reality. So many are ready to revolutionize standards, processes, and systems within the healthcare industry. We truly believe that pharmacists are finding their ways out so that they can come back in.

CHAPTER 5:
CHANGE WILL COME

Unlike some medical professions, pharmacy in general does not have much uniformity or unity in progressing the field into a growing and innovative space. In contrast, nursing has expanded tremendously in its roles over the years, opening up various avenues for practitioners and administrators. Pharmacy's adaptations and expansions are minimal in comparison.

Indeed, clinical opportunities have become available for medication therapy management (MTM) or board certifications, but not all are capable of or desire to land a residency. These roles are exclusionary to most recent graduates or new hires with less experience.

Pharmacy education programs should allow for students to focus on continuous quality improvement courses and certifications. These would include subjects like project management, program management, lean six sigma, health informatics, and other analytics.

Visionaries who want to bring about these changes must be involved in pharmacy administrative programs, education programs, boards, or leadership roles. They must be involved within healthcare reform to highlight the concerns of outcast pharmacists while ensuring proactive change.

Curricula and courses for PharmD programs should begin teaching students what takes place in an actual retail, community, and/or clinical settings day-to-day. Suggestive training shall be provided during educational programs to educate its pharmacy candidates as to how the medical doctors or providers and managed care organizations are all connected. Future pharmacists need to know how significantly these parties impact pharmacies and pharmacy services.

For example:

- *Process prescription insurance.* This is not mentioned with much importance during educational years, despite its importance for outpatient retail/community pharmacists.
- *Preferred pharmacies.* The managed care/insurance companies should be required to display their preferred pharmacies. Student pharmacists need to know what payors have selected as their preferred pharmacy, since it often changes.

As women of faith, we believe that outcast pharmacists will emerge in various fields, unapologetically rejecting the status quo. Our gifts will make room for us, allowing opportunities to continuously come forth. There will be so many opportunities arising for outcasts that we will have to wisely manage our commitments.

Opportunities will arise in our lives where we will not be limited to our physical home addresses, state of residence, or zip codes to determine if we are eligible to fit in a specific professional role. After experiencing the events that have occurred at the beginning of 2020 and throughout 2021 due to the COVID-19 pandemic, pharmacists and healthcare professionals have recognized that many things must change. There has to be a change in order to sustain the profession of pharmacy. Most importantly, change will keep more patients alive and healthy.

Peace is on the horizon for pharmacists, and it will surpass all understanding. For the outcast pharmacist, you will experience joy in fulfilling your purpose in every facet of your life. This will not be due to your degree or your professional pursuits but it will come from the unwavering power of truth.

We as the outcasts will be appreciated for our medical expertise and advocacy roles in protecting patient care, services, and outcomes while working in tandem with other healthcare professionals. We will no longer have to work understaffed or be stretched thin by innumerable tasks and nearly impossible standards.

More roles to hire numerous employees (pharmacists) will come forth because of our defined skill sets, caliber of critical thinking, and trained eye for problem-solving. Our skills will be applied to expanded roles offering salaries commensurate with our education and expertise.

It soon will no longer be difficult to enter into various industries with this specialized professional degree. Training and education may be shortened as well. Several institutions are moving towards a fast-track online matriculation. Our hope is that we will all get paid what we are worth, but at least a comfortable six-figure salary and somewhat of an introductory luxurious net-worth.

Healthcare as we know it will continue to transform over the next five, ten, fifteen years and beyond. Technology will bring about rapid innovation in infrastructure and day-to-day operations of the industry. Advanced technologies and software will decrease human errors and medication discrepancies. Organizations resistant to these changes will fall behind and possibly destruct, if the proper investments are not made to ensure longevity.

This is not to argue that humans can no longer rely on brain power or memory to do such tasks. It is true, however, that humans certainly can and do make errors when fatigued, hungry, or another basic need is unmet. The likelihood of mistakes is heightened even more when repetitive duties are a part of our daily routines.

In essence, health information technology (HIT) needs to become fully interoperable and patient medication awareness must improve dramatically. We believe that, someday in our lifetime, the process of picking up and refilling prescriptions will be similar to depositing money and withdrawing money from ATMs.

Finally, we want to reiterate that this book is intended to be used as a catalyst for change. As we have grown in our faith, we understand the importance and power of writing. Our writing will live longer than we will. We know the skills and assets that pharmacists can provide if the healthcare industry begins recognizing outcast pharmacists.

We have never fit neatly into the box that society and the healthcare industry created for us. We will continue to advocate for the advancement of pharmacists' well-being and for expanding career opportunities. We hope that you too will be a part of these changes and advancements that we desire to see. We invite you to share our message with current and aspiring pharmacists. Your support and encouragement will mean more to them than you know.

REFERENCES

"Alert fatigue or alarm fatigue." Merriam-Webster Dictionary.
https://www.merriam-webster.com/dictionary/alertfatigue

American Pharmacists Association (2021). "Career Option Profiles." https://www.pharmacist.com/career-option-profiles

"Distress." Merriam-Webster Dictionary. https://www.merriam-webster.com/dictionary/distress

"Eating disorders." Merriam-Webster Dictionary. https://www.merriam-webster.com/dictionary/eatingdisorders

"Emotionally exhausted." Merriam-Webster Dictionary. https://www.merriam-webster.com/dictionary/emotionallyexhausted

"Job burnout or occupational burnout." Merriam-Webster Dictionary. https://www.merriam-webster.com/dictionary/jobburnnout

"Outcast." Merriam-Webster Dictionary. https://www.merriam-webster.com/dictionary/outcast

"Overworked." Merriam-Webster Dictionary. https://www.merriam-webster.com/dictionary/overworked

"Pharmacist." Merriam-Webster Dictionary. https://www.merriam-webster.com/dictionary/pharmacist

"Pharmacy intern." Florida Legislature Statues Index. http://www.leg.state.fl.us/Statutes/index.cfm?App_mode=Display_Statute&URL=0400-0499/0465/Sections/0465.003.html

"Physical, physiological, and psychological distress." Merriam-Webster Dictionary. https://www.merriam-webster.com/dictionary/physiologicaldistress

"Regret." Merriam-Webster Dictionary. https://www.merriam-webster.com/dictionary/regret

"Understaffed." https://www.merriam-webster.com/dictionary/understaffed

ABOUT THE AUTHORS

Dr. Amber Goodman and Dr. Ashley Goodman are known for their unique and tailored writing styles of concise yet impactful, easily digestible, and detailed content for their target audiences. Drs. Amber and Ashley are a dynamic duo of emerging young leaders, evangelists, and college professors. Their church home for spiritual training and equipping is Heaven to Earth Worship Center, Tampa, FL.

As a result of their upbringing, academics and athletics have molded these two into the leaders they are today. Both received full scholarships to play basketball in addition to receiving academic scholarships. After basketball concluded, their vision was set to become doctors of pharmacy. Their faith in Jesus Christ, along with a love for the apostolic and prophetic, has led them to accept the call as five-fold ministers and to further their education within the fields of public health and business administration.

As growing figureheads in healthcare with a passion for full-time ministry, they are determined to influence the quality of healthcare delivery and systems for generations to come. With this spiritual mandate, both aspire to bring light to those who are in darkness, helping others discover salvation and their place in God's perfect will. Doctors Ashley and Amber plan to continue imparting revelations of the Lord through the spirits of knowledge, wisdom, and counsel.

ACKNOWLEDGMENTS

We acknowledge our Lord and Savior Jesus Christ; our lovely parents, Dr. Carl B. Goodman & Jacqueline Goodman; our spiritual parents and Overseer, Prophet Daniel Powell, Sr. & Prophetess Esther Powell; Faith and Works Outreach International Ministries; and Heaven to Earth Worship Center located in Tampa, FL.

Made in the USA
Middletown, DE
11 April 2022

64028176R00022